The First Cry

Understanding Why Babies Cry At Birth And For The First 12 Months.

By

Helen R. Howard

CONTENTS

Introduction

The First Cry

About The Baby's First Cry.

Importance Of Baby's First Cry.

First Minutes After Baby Is Born

Characteristics of the first cry

The benefits of the first cry for mother and baby

How Your Baby Will Look And Behave After Birth.

What if your Newborn Doesn't Cry at Birth?

The science behind crying

Why Do Babies Cry?

Are there certain times of the day when my baby will cry more?

How To Cope With Uncontrollable Crying

The First Cry.

Busting the crying myths

Will my baby's crying change as they grow?

How to relieve your baby's crying

Conclusion

Introduction

Probably one of the most rewarding jobs you'll ever have is becoming a parent. Additionally, it ranks among the hardest. You'll understand that you're entitled to a break occasionally after adding a few hours of crying to the mix.

Try to periodically let someone else (your partner, a member of your family, or a friend) take charge. Take a shower or go for a walk with the time. Even better, lie up in bed, look through your collection of baby photos, and tell yourself once more that you're the best parent for your kid.

Chapter 1

The First Cry

The first cry of the newborn infant announces the beginning of a brand-new, independent life. It is vociferous, shrill, and piercing. The cry of a newborn serves as a request for protection, care, and support after being cut off from the mother's body. However, what does the initial cry convey? Or is the cry just a form of expression? What potential meaning could the cry have? Although we might be able to explain the cry's purpose, we are perplexed by the mystery of its meaning. The physiognomy and genesis of the first cry are added to the first cry's scientific understanding in this study. It poses the question of how, in light of what is known about embryology, neonatology, and related medical research, the primordial inequality and elemental sensibility of the first cry may be qualitatively probed and comprehended. The phenomenological physiology of a newborn's first cry compels us to make cautious assumptions about its implications for health sciences, adults, and children.

Despite the fact that the majority of newborns are delivered head first, they are unable to breathe once their heads have emerged because their chests are still under too much pressure. Your infant's respiratory reflex begins to function once you deliver the baby and the pressure subsides.

Your little one will cough or sputter as they expel the fluid that is blocking their airway and fill their lungs with air. As the air speeds past their vocal cords, voila, that first cry rings out.

Recent studies suggest that examining these early crying patterns may help distinguish between newborns with healthy lungs and those who have respiratory distress syndrome.

Enjoy your baby's first beautiful cries as they indicate that their respiratory and circulatory systems are successfully adapting to life outside of your womb.

Because they are startled by the transfer to the outside world, newborns may continue to wail. Breastfeeding and skin-to-skin contact will provide them with the solace they need.

About The Baby's First Cry.

You've already seen how important it is to understand the cause of a baby's cry, both immediately and later. We must not lose sight of the fact that this is their sole means of communication, both to request assistance and to express their emotions. The first cry, in particular, is crucial for the baby's adjustment to the extrauterine environment and has numerous positive effects on both the mother and the baby's health.

Simply said, the body is extremely intelligent, and everything that occurs naturally serves a function. In this instance, nature makes sure that the little one who has recently entered our lives and is about to completely transform them receives all of our attention.

Importance Of Baby's First Cry.

The joy of hearing your Baby's First Cry is almost an indescribable feeling. Why is it so important to hear your baby cry within the first minute of birth?

As you progress in your motherhood, the incessant crying of your baby might leave you irritated to no end. But the first cry is always the most joyous moment of a mother's life. This assures the doctor as well that your baby has ticked one of the most important signs for survival.

During your baby's stay in the womb, the umbilical cord carries oxygen and carbon dioxide from the placenta into your baby's bloodstream. As soon as your baby is born, it should begin crying within the first 30 seconds to one minute of life, his/ her first cry will be at the top of your doctor's priority list. The reason is, your baby's first cry acts as a kick-starter for their little lungs, as it helps them to get rid of any amniotic residue and other secretions in the lungs and nasal passages.

When a baby doesn't cry or start breathing right away after birth, it is regarded as a medical emergency. A baby who is unable to breathe cannot develop an independent life separate from its mother and must undergo neonatal resuscitation, which simply means that the baby needs some kind of help to start breathing.

The first cry, therefore, denotes a smooth shift from "breathing" fluid in the womb to breathing air after birth. As the infant's nervous system adjusts to the sudden shift in environment and temperature, it emits a breath that sounds like a gasp.

A variety of modifications to the infant's lungs and circulatory system take place once the first breath is taken:

Lung blood flow resistance decreases when oxygen levels in the lungs rise.

The baby's blood vessels blood flow resistance also rises.

From the respiratory system, amniotic fluid either drains or is absorbed.

The lungs expand and start functioning on their own, supplying the bloodstream with oxygen and eliminating carbon dioxide through exhaling (exhalation).

You now realize that your baby's first cry is akin to their first breath and may even be their method of introducing themselves to you and the outside world.

First Minutes After Baby Is Born

There may be a lot going on during the time of your baby's birth, but it can also be a really memorable moment. Depending on your labor, how your baby is delivered, and how fast your infant adjusts to life outside the womb, what happens immediately after birth will vary.

Uncomplicated vaginal birth

Most babies breathe and cry within a few seconds of being born.

Immediately after birth, if your baby is breathing OK, you can place him or her on your chest or belly, naked and next to you. Skin-to-skin contact helps you and your newborn form an immediate physical bond while keeping your infant warm and regulating their breathing and heart rate. Additionally, breastfeeding is triggered by it.

While your infant is on you, the midwife will dry him or her, then she will wrap you both in a warm blanket or towel.

Forceps or vacuum birth

Most babies delivered using forceps or a vacuum will breathe and cry when they are born. However, some infants may appear dazed or have trouble breathing, particularly if their mothers were disturbed when giving birth. The midwife, obstetrician, or pediatrician will take your child to a designated warming station if this occurs. They will dry your child and monitor their respiration.

Once your kid is breathing normally, you can hold him or her. Requesting skin-to-skin contact is an option. Alternatively, your infant can be cleaned and wrapped in warm blankets or towels for you to hold.

Elective cesarean section

The majority of newborns delivered by elective c-section breathe and cry a lot right after birth.

Before the baby is taken to a special warming station to be dried and assessed, if the infant is breathing normally, you might be able to touch him or her on the skin. Before returning the infant to your care, its breathing may occasionally be checked. If you like, the baby can be wrapped in warm blankets or towels and placed in your arms while you are on the operation table, or you can ask to hold your child skin-to-skin.

Sometimes you could require additional medical care, so your first hug might have to wait. Until you return to recovery or the maternity ward, your birth partner can stay with your infant and provide plenty of cuddling and skin-to-skin contact.

Unplanned (emergency) cesarean section

Unplanned cesarean births increase the risk of newborns needing assistance breathing. Your infant will be sent to an exclusive warming station by the midwife or pediatrician so that it can dry off. They will also look into the kind of assistance your child requires.

The First Cry.

You can hold your kid after they're breathing normally and you're feeling fine. It's acceptable to request skin-to-skin contact or cuddling while you're still on the surgical table.

You will be allowed to hold your baby once you've recovered if you underwent a general anesthetic.

Characteristics of the first cry

The characteristics of a baby's first wail do not elevate it above or below other first cries in terms of normalcy. Each infant does it in a unique way, and I'll explain what it means to you:

The infant's wail is piercing and loud. In general, healthy babies cry a lot when they are first born as a result of the aforementioned adaptation process. It merely describes the stress brought on by a rapid shift in environment and doesn't necessarily imply pain or discomfort.

When a newborn cries passively yet effectively, it may indicate that the baby was comfortable and sleepy when it emerged from the womb. This is frequently the case with scheduled cesarean sections because there is almost no need for the patient's participation in the delivery process. The normalcy of the remaining Apgar scale criteria will determine how the next kind differs.

The baby either doesn't cry at all or cries very little. This could be a sign of an insufficient ability to adjust to the extrauterine environment due to a lack of pulmonary maturity or birth or gestational problem. In this situation, it is important to evaluate the youngster very away and provide any necessary assistance.

The benefits of the first cry for mother and baby

Although we concentrated on the effects of the first cry's qualities on the baby's physical health in the preceding sections, they are not just confined to that. In reality, the mother also gains from it. Here are some of its primary advantages:

It assists in clearing the airways of any amniotic fluid that may be present.

It encourages the start of the infant's respiratory activity.

It aids in the body of the infant's changing circulatory system (transition from fetal to neonatal circulation).

It provides the mother with a variety of psychological advantages, including promoting the release of chemicals necessary for the development of attachment and brings peace and relief during childbirth.

Oxytocin, a crucial hormone for uterine contraction and the start of lactation, is produced as a result of it.

Crying is also a way to communicate

Crying happens for a variety of physiological reasons as well as a means of communication between the newborn and its environment. The baby can only communicate through crying if it is scared, anxious, in pain, hungry, or in need of affection.

The sound of the infant crying instinctively sets off a number of responses in the mother's brain. There has been numerous research on infant crying, and some intriguing conclusions have been made:

Even if people who are seeing a newborn cry might not understand why the baby is crying, their brain reacts more when they believe the crying to be a sign of pain than when they believe it to be a sign of fear or anger.

Babies' eyes are open as they cry out in fear or rage. However, they basically keep them closed when the cause is discomfort.

Infants who cry more and more frequently with time typically do so out of rage or displeasure. Contrarily, crying brought on by pain or anxiety begins intensely and continues to be so.

Chapter 2

How Your Baby Will Look And Behave After Birth.

Your infant may appear blue or purple in the first few minutes after birth; this is typical. Within 7 to 10 minutes of birth, if your baby is breathing normally, the hue of the skin will progressively turn pink. The hands and feet of your infant could remain blue for up to 24 hours. This is due to the fact that the blood arteries in your baby's hands and feet are so tiny that it takes some time for the blood to circulate normally and cause the tissues to turn pink.

Most newborns cry right away after birth if everything goes OK. The majority then quietly observe their surroundings while keeping their eyes wide open before nodding off. But some people might continue to be awake and crave food.

Within a few minutes of giving delivery, you can try nursing if your infant seems ready. The midwife will assist you in nursing the infant.

Below are a few looks and behaviors of your newborn;

1. **Skin-to-skin contact**

   Your newborn baby will be placed on your chest for skin-to-skin contact following a typical vaginal birth. Your infant needs to feel your skin in order to get the rest and nourishment they require as well as to feel safe and warm.

   They will be weighed, measured, and observed after this initial interaction to make sure they are in good health.

   Ask your midwife to ensure that your baby has skin-to-skin contact with you as soon as possible if you have a cesarean section. In the operating room and afterward, you or your spouse might be able to hold your infant skin-to-skin.

2. Feeding

Soon after delivery, babies begin to exhibit signs of hunger, and they typically connect to and suck at the breast approximately 50 minutes later. They may continue nursing for an hour or longer after that. If you place your infant against your chest, they will likely start nursing from your breast. Ask your midwife or a lactation consultant for assistance if that doesn't work.

Colostrum is the name for the first milk you produce. Instead of being pure white, it is thick and frequently yellowish. This milk is perfect for your infant. Your baby's belly typically only produces a tiny amount, about the size of a marble.

Try again a few hours later if they haven't fed within an hour or two of birth.

3. Sleeping

Your infant will remain with you so that you may get to know them and meet their needs quickly. After their first feeding, they'll generally fall asleep shortly, and they might sleep for around six hours. More than likely, they will spend the majority of their first day in the world sleeping.

4. Hearing.

Your baby will recognize your voice when you speak to them after birth because they have been listening to it for the second half of your pregnancy. If your partner or another support person has been conversing close to your kid, you might recognize their voice as well. When your baby hears your words, they will feel secure and may react by tilting their head in your direction. The same as when they were in the womb, your kid will be able to hear your heartbeat.

5. Vision

Although your baby's vision is blurry at birth, they can focus on your face from a distance of about 30 centimeters. This is referred to as the "cuddle distance." It generally equates to the space between your breast and your face. Your child will establish a connection between what they hear and see.

6. Urine and meconium

Your infant will likely urinate and pass meconium (newborn feces) at least once during the first 24 hours. Meconium has a dark, sticky color. Over the coming days, the color and consistency of your baby's poop will vary.

Does my baby recognize me?

Your newborn will like your face over that of a stranger shortly after birth, and he or she might even smile at you!

Your infant also recognizes you by smell, according to their sense of smell. You are providing your baby with the chance to develop more accustomed to your distinctive odors while you are nursing or otherwise in close proximity to your youngster. Babies are able to distinguish between the smells of their mother and either unfamiliar breastfeeding women or women who have never given birth, according to research. The smell of your mother is one that newborns start to love, and it may even be able to calm or comfort your child.

If you're a new parent, you might be concerned that your child doesn't recognize you yet or that you won't be able to tell when they do. Keep in mind that every infant is different and that they will each acquire preferences at a different rate. It could also take some time for you to become familiar with your baby's cues and behaviors. They will continually be exposed to your voices and faces over the next few months, giving them the chance to get to know you better. Spend some quality time with your new baby now.

Chapter 3

What if your Newborn Doesn't Cry at Birth?

There have been numerous occasions where a baby has been born and not cried. However, when you really see it, it can come as quite a shock because it would indicate that your baby is not breathing.

Your baby's cry is a sign that his or her lungs are healthy enough for breathing. If your kid doesn't cry right away, there's probably no need to be alarmed. Many newborns are healthy when they are born, pink and alert with all of their limbs moving, and they may not cry for several minutes. In cases where the baby's hue is not a healthy pink and there are indications of a struggle, doctors are aware of this and do take additional steps. To remove any impediments from the road, the suction pump is used speedily. Although many doctors also choose to massage the baby, the traditional technique of spanking the baby is only performed as a last option to inflict some pain and make it cry aloud. The infant is sent to the intensive care unit (ICU) and artificial oxygen supply tubes are employed to provide the body with oxygen if all of these treatments fail as well.

The medical staff can verify a baby's lungs are healthy by listening to their cry upon birth. It's common for parents to hear doctors compliment a newborn's cry, but does this imply that a kid who doesn't cry at delivery is less healthy?

The science behind crying

There are other non-vocal aspects of weeping in addition to the distinctive sound that babies make when they cry. Despite the fact that crying appears to be a pretty simple activity, it actually requires the synchronization of a number of intricate parts, including the face's muscles, airways, and respiratory system.

The non-vocal components of crying actually start to emerge in the womb, according to a 2005 study. In the study, 10 fetuses in the womb were exposed to vibroacoustic stimulation, which involves administering a sound and vibration stimulus to the mother's belly. As a response, all of the fetuses displayed fetal weeping behavior. They displayed breathing patterns that resembled post-womb sobbing, and they frowned or grimaced while still in the womb. The research concluded that the fetus possesses all of the motor skill coordination required for the non-vocal component of weeping by the time it is 20 weeks gestation.

Crying directly after birth

When a baby is delivered, they are exposed to a new environment and chilly air, which frequently causes them to cry right away. The baby's lungs will grow during this cry, and amniotic fluid and mucus will be released. The infant's first actual cry confirms that the lungs are functioning normally. However, a number of various circumstances, such as a challenging delivery, a nuchal cord, etc., could cause the cry to be postponed.

When to worry

It's not always a sign that a baby is unwell if its cry is delayed. If the infant's first cry does not come naturally, your doctor may try to elicit it by drying the baby off or sucking fluid from their mouth or nose.

The infant needs to receive rapid medical care if a delayed cry is accompanied by additional emergency symptoms. Measurements are made using the Apgar scale for these additional aspects of a newborn baby's examination. score.

The parts of the Apgar score are:

A – Appearance (skin color)

P – Pulse (heart rate)

G – Grimace (reflex irritability/response)

A – Activity (muscle tone)

R – Respiration (breathing ability)

Each of the five criteria is scored from 0 to 2 (two being the best), and the sum of all five scores gives the final score. An Apgar test will often be performed by your doctor one and five minutes following the birth. If the initial score is low, a second Apgar test may be administered at 10, 15, and 20 minutes.

The severity of the required intervention can be determined by the scores.

A score of:

0-3 baby is in critical condition

4-6 baby likely needs immediate medical intervention

7-10 baby is within normal range but should still be monitored

Though a score above 7 is considered normal, a recent study showed that Apgar scores of 7-9 could still be associated with adverse outcomes. A score below 10 should still be monitored, even if it's in the 7-10 range.

Chapter 4.

Why Do Babies Cry?

Most likely, a cry is the first indication that your baby had arrived. It was a joy to hear, and you embraced it with wide ears, whether it was a full-throated wail, a delicate bleat, or a string of desperate screams.

Now when it has been days, weeks, or even months, you are reaching for the earplugs. When will your infant stop sobbing?

Although expectant parents know their baby will grumble and cry, nothing will prepare you for what seems like unending, unrelenting crying. Let's explore the meaning behind your baby's screams and squalls, as well as how to calm them down so that everyone may enjoy some well-deserved tranquility.

Common causes of crying

In infants 3 months and younger

Your infant has many important things to tell you. In the first several months of life, they may be crying because they:

- **Have Digestive issues**

   The digestive system of your kid is growing, and this involves a lot of learning. Every step can be a cause for tears until everything runs properly.

- **Are Hungry**

   The most frequent cause of crying in infants is hunger. Thankfully, taking care of it is simple. Your infant will relax once they begin to eat. Unless the item after that on our list starts.

You can hold them upright under the arms while supporting the head, drape them across your arm, or put them over your shoulder. Have a burp cloth on hand to mop up any spittle.

- **Have Dirty diapers**

Verify that the diaper on your child is clean. Their delicate skin will become irritated by poop, especially if they already have a rash. Every time you change their diaper, spread some diaper cream over the region to prevent problems.

Too late? Diaper rash can be healed with a milk bath. According to a 2013 study, utilizing breast milk to cure diaper rash is just as efficient as using hydrocortisone 1% ointment by itself.

- **Have Food sensitivities and allergies**

Know that whatever you consume gets transferred to your kid through your milk if you breastfeed. Dairy, gluten, and eggs can all be challenging for your infant to digest.

Rarely do young children have true food sensitivities. However, you might want to change your diet if you're nursing. If your baby is formula-fed, discuss changing formulas with your healthcare professional.

At six months, solid foods are often offered. You should discuss when to introduce common allergens including cow's milk, peanuts, seafood, wheat, and eggs with your healthcare professional. Depending on whether your child is at a high risk of having a food allergy, this schedule may change. Your doctor is the best person to advise you on this.

- **Are fatigued.**

Babies who are awake for an excessive amount of time or who are overstimulated may get overtired. Your infant will cry, yawn, touch or pull at their ears, cling to you, or get disoriented as an indication that they are sleepy. At this moment, your task is to put them to sleep.

Swaddling, feeding, rocking, providing a pacifier, and dimming the environment are all things to try. Laying your infant on their back in their bed or bassinet will help them fall asleep.

- **Are Running temperature**

Just like us, newborns dislike extreme temperatures. To check if your baby's onesie is damp from perspiration, run your finger along the back of it. Check to see if your baby's ears are too cold by touching them. Dress them appropriately after that.

- are alone or bored
- have eaten too much (causing a bloated stomach)
- need to poop or urinate
- need affection or comfort
- are too stimulated by activity or noise
- are annoyed by clothing that is rough or a tag
- need to be swaddled or rocked

Are you shocked that intestinal gas is not included on the list? According to the American Academy of Pediatrics, a baby's lower digestive system experiencing gas is not uncomfortable. You would assume that the fact that they are letting out a lot of gas when they cry is the source of their anguish, however, it is a fallacy that gas gets caught in the intestines and causes pain.

In babies older than 3 months

The physiological reasons for a newborn's crying, like hunger, depending on the parent's ability to comfort them.

Babies who are more than 3 or 4 months old have probably acquired the art of utilizing their thumb, fist, or pacifier to soothe themselves. However, it doesn't mean they don't occasionally break into song. They may be expressing their frustration, sadness, anger, or separation anxiety through sobbing (particularly at night). They may also be expressing their sadness or separation anxiety.

Older babies' sobbing is frequently brought on by the pain of teething. Most infants begin to erupt their first tooth between the ages of 6 and 12. Your infant may be fussy and cry, as well as have swollen and sore gums and drool more frequently than usual.

Offer your kid a fresh, chilled, or wet towel or a sturdy teething ring to ease the pain of teething. Consult your pediatrician about administering an adequate amount of acetaminophen if the weeping persists (Tylenol). If your child is older than six months, you can also give them ibuprofen (Advil).

Are there certain times of the day when my baby will cry more?

Indeed, there are. The "witching hour" refers to the times of day when your infant is most prone to cry. Your kid will generally have the most trouble sleeping between the hours of 5 p.m. and 12 a.m.

When your kid is between two and three weeks old, these tough hours start. Fortunately, they stop around the time your baby turns three months old.

There is no clear explanation for why these predictable fussy spells occur, although the majority of medical professionals concur that a full day of stimulation and a reduction in the mother's milk supply at night are major factors.

Actually, not every newborn baby cries upon taking their first breath. But if they are not instantly joined with their mother, all infants will start to wail within a few seconds. This straightforward modification lessens the likelihood that they will be forgotten.

In fact, there is considerable evidence that suggests that baby screams have expressly developed to be as inconvenient and difficult to ignore as possible. Neonatal infants may wail for the first few minutes after delivery and during their first feeding since the trauma of giving birth has left them wounded and painful, but often they will fall asleep for the next eight hours or so.

Chapter 5

How To Cope With Uncontrollable Crying

Once more, you're rocking a baby who is wailing and wishing you were somewhere else. How can you handle this? Inhale the divine aroma by placing your nose in the tender area of your infant's neck. Next, try these strategies:

Become calm. All right, so it's easier said than done. It's worth the work, though. Promise. How come it works? We are wired to synchronize with an outside rhythm; this process is known as entrainment. Therefore, your kid will naturally mimic your breathing and heartbeat when breathing and beating. Keep them moving slowly.

Cluster feed. Your infant might require a nursing session every 30 minutes or more throughout the witching hour. That's totally OK. Cluster feeding will perhaps help them feel fuller so they can sleep through the night for extended periods of time.

Use a pacifier. All infants have a strong desire to suckle. Instead of giving your infant your breast or a bottle to relax them, you may try giving them a pacifier. Along with calming your infant, sucking will also aid in the digestion of the milk already present in their stomach thanks to all the saliva they ingest.

Allow for skin-to-skin contact. Holding your infant to your chest while they are completely naked allows them to hear your heartbeat and can help calm them.

Do a tourniquet syndrome check. Inspect your baby to make sure the hair hasn't gotten caught around his or her fingers, toes, or genitalia. The hair may restrict blood flow, resulting in edema and redness. Though it's quite uncommon, keep a watch out.

When the fussiness is long term

Here are a few things you might look into if your infant appears to be sobbing uncontrollably often:

Reflux

Your baby may sob uncontrollably if they have gastroesophageal reflux disease (GERD). You may be dealing with reflux if your baby frequently spits up large amounts, is excessively wiggly during or after feedings, or becomes predictably fussy when lying on their back.

Regurgitated stomach acids that irritate the esophagus are known as reflux. By recalling how heartburn feels, you can empathize with your infant.

In order to self-soothe and alleviate heartburn, babies with reflux frequently feel the urge to suck. However, if reflux is the cause of their fussiness and they eat more, it could exacerbate the reflux. Offer a pacifier to your baby before overfeeding if you think reflux is the source of their discomfort.

Colic

Baby cries caused by colic are unusual. If your infant cries for three or more hours a day, three or more days a week, for three weeks, your pediatrician will diagnose your child with colic.

Colic often begins when your kid is six weeks old and finishes in the third or fourth month. Your best chance of surviving this incredibly difficult stage is to become an expert at the swaddle, side-stomach position, shush, swing, and suck.

Pain

You'll be able to identify a cry of agony as you learn to decipher your baby's cries. An urgent, high-pitched wail is typically used to indicate agony.

Pain is experienced when one has an earache, a mouth ulcer, or a diaper rash. For a diagnosis, speak with your doctor. Call your doctor if your infant develops a fever and is younger than three months old.

Busting the crying myths

We've all heard that crying helps a baby's lungs develop. It has a strong hold on our psyche, just like all myths do. The question is, though, if it's accurate.

Nope. In actuality, this claim is unsupported by any research. But a wealth of data demonstrates that moms who act immediately and consistently in the face of their infants' cries are teaching their young charges that "Yes, you matter, and what you want is essential to me."

To prevent your child from becoming spoilt and needing to be scooped up constantly, well-meaning family and friends may urge you to ignore your baby's cries. Avoid them. There is no such thing as spoiling a newborn, according to experts.

Will my baby's crying change as they grow?

The feeding, age, surroundings, and temperament of a newborn all have an effect on their behavior. All newborns experience variations in their crying patterns, and sometimes it can be challenging to figure out why.

When they transition into a new developmental stage, babies also alter their sleeping and feeding schedules. The same holds true for times when kids are ill, teething, or anxious about being separated.

Babies need constant, compassionate care to feel safe during the first three years of life as they are building connections or pathways in their brains. Parents, who frequently feel exhausted and sleep deprived, must expend a lot of energy on this.

Your baby's sleep patterns will become more predictable as they become older. On a 24-hour day, a newborn sleeps for between 14 and 17 hours. They will require less sleep during the day as they become older and more sleep at night.

How to relieve your baby's crying

Here are the things to try if you have an inconsolable little one:

Feed your baby

With this one, you should try to be a little proactive. It's likely that you performed this right away when your infant started crying, but it could not have had the desired effect. Sometimes, when sobbing becomes more intense, offering the breast or a bottle causes frenetic and haphazard sucking.

"You're already running behind schedule if a baby starts screaming out of hunger.

Keep an eye out for these signs that your child is starting to grow hungry: When they frantically dig around for the nipple or suck on their hands is one sign. Offer the breast or bottle while they are still peaceful to avoid unrelenting sobbing and the frenzied, frequently unsuccessful feeding that follows.

Identify your baby's cries

A sudden, prolonged, high-pitched screech typically implies pain, but a quick, low-pitched, rising-and-falling cry usually signifies hunger. It is impossible to generalize what a specific cry implies to all babies, though.

From baby to baby, crying differs and is greatly influenced by temperament. You could wonder if there's something wrong with them if your previous child was quite laid-back and this new baby is, well, not so much.

There is probably nothing wrong; some newborns simply have more sensitive temperaments and express themselves in more spectacular ways when they cry.

If you watch and listen to your baby every day, you'll soon be able to identify the various cries they make. If your baby cries when they are hungry, pay attention to how it sounds and how it differs from other cries.

Imagine that you are studying a new language to aid. (Believe me.) If you actually pay attention to your baby's cries, you and the child will eventually come up with your own lexicon.

Notice your baby's 'tells'

There are other, more subdued signs that hint at what your baby needs exist, and recognizing them will help you avoid crying fits.

Some of these are obvious, like when someone yawns or rubs their eyes when they're fatigued.

Others are less evident, like turning away from the stimulus when they've had enough of it. To learn these signs, pay close attention to your baby's movements, positions, facial expressions, and vocal sounds (like as whimpering) throughout the day.

Keep in mind that each infant is special. Your second child won't necessarily suck on your hand when they're hungry just because your first did. This behavior may be interpreted as "I need to calm down."

Put yourself in their place

If your baby's cry or other indications don't reveal what is upsetting him or her, consider what would annoy you if you were the one who was upset. The TV is it too loud? Is the overhead illumination too strong? Do you ever get bored? Afterward, take the necessary action.

Your baby will likely benefit from a change of environment if you carry them about in a front-facing carrier or take them outdoors in a stroller if you fear they are getting bored.

Provide relaxing white noise by turning on a fan or the clothes dryer to drown out background noise in the house and imitate the shushing your baby experienced while still in the womb.

Consider other relief strategies

If crying still has no apparent cause, try these things:

cradling the infant in your arms or a chair (rapid tiny movements generally are best for calming)

Sweating your infant (ask your pediatrician or nurse how or check out our how-to)

giving them a warm bath, swinging them, and singing to them

Check hands, feet, and genitalia for "hair tourniquets" (a hair tightly wrapped around a finger, toe, or penis), which can definitely set off your infant, if you think your kid is in discomfort.

Do one thing at a time

Parents frequently employ several different tactics in short succession in an effort to put an end to the wailing.

"Parents typically hold, bounce, shush, sing, pat, and change postures all at once! Additionally, they will attempt to change the diaper, feed, and then hand the child off to the other parent for a turn. Frequently, all of them occur in a matter of minutes. The only effect of this is to overstimulate the infant.

Instead, perform one activity at a time, such as just singing, just rocking, or just patting, and persist with it for about five minutes to observe whether your baby calms down. If not, consider a different pain-relief strategy.

Address the colic

If your doctor verifies that your baby has colic, keep in mind that it has nothing to do with how you are parenting.

I advise you to try a special infant massage designed for colicky newborns to lessen the crying. It promotes relaxation, sleep, digestion, and a strong link between you and your child.

For on-the-spot massages for colic, there are YouTube videos. Alternatively, you can find a baby massage expert who can show you how to assist your colicky child.

Just let them cry (within reason)

Your infant gets fed and diapered. They've bounced, rocked, been petted, and listened to songs. You're worn out, irritated, and overburdened. Every parent of a newborn has experienced it.

Put your infant in a secure location, such as their crib, and leave the room if you're on the verge of losing it.

One possibility is to ask your spouse, a member of your family, or a close friend to take charge. If it's not, understand that allowing your child to "cry it out" for a little period of time won't have any long-term negative effects.

"We are aware that occasionally letting newborns scream does not emotionally harm them. This topic has undergone much research. By how much? Your baby may need to cry in order to change from a waking to a sleeping state, and you may feel okay about letting her do so in the long run, depending on both you and your baby. This is especially true if you are near your emotional breaking point.

But when you're at your wit's end, trying to calm your wailing baby much longer could have long-term consequences. When a sleep-deprived, irrational parent can no longer tolerate the wailing, shaken baby syndrome frequently results.

Take a deep breath, take a short break, and remember that parenting is challenging when you feel at your breaking point.

How do I look after myself when my baby is crying?

It's crucial to take care of your personal needs because parenting can sometimes feel more like a marathon than a sprint. This entails having consistent, wholesome meals, drinking plenty of water, getting as much relaxation and sleep as you can, and understanding when to ask for assistance. Accept any acceptable support that is offered to you by your loved ones.

Though your baby is upset, try to maintain your composure. Do some breathing exercises and mindfulness exercises.

Recognize that you won't always be able to predict what your baby wants. Try to perceive their sobbing as their main form of communication rather than something you need to "correct."

What are the signs my baby is unwell?

Take your baby to a doctor if they have:

- a fever of more than 38 degrees Celsius,
- vomiting, diarrhea
- trouble breathing, a rash, or pale or blue skin,
- changes in their feeding schedule,
- less wet or dirty diapers.

Additionally, you shouldn't be reluctant to take your infant to the doctor if you have any concerns or think that something is wrong.

Avoid these mistakes when your baby is crying

When your kid is crying, especially when you can't get them to stop, it can be stressful and distressing at times.

What's important is that you never:

Shake your infant, this can result in bleeding in the brain, which can result in death or severe brain damage.

raise your voice, hit them, or otherwise act out your rage toward your infant. Approximately

When you are angry, remain physically near your child.

Put your kid in their cot and leave if you see that your own crying is becoming overwhelming. When you feel peaceful, come back. Keep an eye on your own mental health, and if you start to feel nervous or depressed, consult your doctor or a child health nurse.

Conclusion

You might think it's impossible right now, but eventually, the crying fits will stop.

A 2017 study found that during the first few weeks after birth, newborns cry for about two hours per day. By 6 weeks, the crying has increased and peaked at 2 to 3 hours each day. Thereafter, it gradually declines (hallelujah!). A baby's weeping will generally total no more than an hour per day by the time they are 4 months old.

Even more comforting: By that time, you will have accumulated a great deal of knowledge about how to recognize your baby's cues and screams, so attending to their needs should stop the uncontrollable sobbing that characterized their early weeks. You can do this.